Mastering Emotions:

A Practical Manual for Managing Your Feelings and Overcoming Negativity

By

Mary R. Dalton

TABLE OF CONTENTS

INTRODUCTION

Understanding emotions will help you choose how to react to them in the most effective way, which is one solid reason to do so. In psychology and neuroscience, research on emotion is now a prominent area of growth. It is crucial first to determine whether your feelings match the present scenario before deciding how to react. Understanding emotions may also be beneficial since it might make it easier for you to comprehend others. Maybe you've witnessed someone become upset or outraged in a circumstance, but you couldn't understand why.

Emotional reactions can be beneficial when they occur under the appropriate circumstances. For instance, if a snake makes you nervous, your fear will encourage you to avoid snakes and prevent getting bitten. Or, if you become furious when someone mistreats you, your rage may persuade the offender to stop being cruel. Or, if your loved ones observe your grief in the wake of a friend's departure, they will understand that you require their love and support.

However, these feelings may occasionally be counterproductive if they occur in the wrong circumstances. For instance, your friendship may suffer if you are upset with a buddy because he accidentally wounded you. Or, if you are so terrified of exams that you skip class, this could help prevent you from earning a high mark in that course. Or, if you grieve for too long after a buddy leaves, it could be more difficult for you to meet new people.

They presumably have different life experiences than you have, which is why they perceive the issue differently. Generally speaking, taking any time will probably also help you comprehend why a person feels the way they do if you try to grasp what that person could be thinking and what experiences they may have had in the past.

Exercise and activity are some things that might assist if you are angry or unhappy. For instance, when someone is upset, they frequently desire to shout or say cruel things. But going for a run instead often assists individuals in calming down, improving their ability to think effectively, and elevating their mood.

In another instance, when people are depressed, they frequently just want to sit at home by themselves and reflect on their troubles. They could occasionally feel worse as a result, though. When you're dejected, Even if you don't feel like it, getting outside and exercising may be pretty beneficial. You may, for instance, go out with a buddy or take a stroll in a park.

What is said here is not an attempt to define or explain emotion. The goal is to provide a framework for thinking about certain critical phenomena linked with emotion (phenomena related to survival processes) without being confused by the definition of emotion. The easiest way out of the conceptual impasse that emerges from repeated discussions about what emotion is may be to step back from the overarching notion of emotion and concentrate instead on essential facts that make emotion an intriguing topic.

CHAPTER ONE

Understanding emotions

Emotions have a significant impact on your thoughts and actions. The feelings you experience daily may motivate you to act and affect the big and minor decisions you make about your life.

Emotions can be fleeting, like a flash of irritation at a coworker, or they can be persistent, like everlasting grief at the end of a relationship. But why do we actually feel emotions? What purpose do they fulfill?

Your emotions may spur you to action.

You could worry about how you will do and how the examination will affect your final score before a stressful exam. These feelings may make you more motivated to learn as a result.

You also tend to act in specific ways to increase the likelihood of having happy emotions and decrease the possibility of having negative ones. For instance, you can look for hobbies or social activities that make you feel pleased, content, and energetic. Conversely, you would generally steer clear of any circumstances that would cause boredom, unhappiness, or fear.

Emotions increase your chance of acting. You're more inclined to tackle the cause of your irritation while you're upset. Fear makes you more prone to run away from danger. If you're in love, you could look for a partner.

The Three Elements of Emotions

Understanding the three essential elements of emotion is crucial to fully comprehending it. Each component has a potential impact on the kind and intent of your emotional reactions.

1. Subjective component: Your emotional experience
2. Physical element: Your body's response to the feeling.
3. The expressive component is how you react to the feeling.

4 Reasons Why Emotions Matter

1. Your emotions can help you stay safe.

Emotional outbursts can also be crucial for protection and survival. If you came across an animal hissing or spitting, it would be evident that the animal was enraged and on the defensive, so you should back off and maybe escape harm.

The body might get ready to behave as a result of emotions. The amygdala is mainly responsible for setting off emotional reactions that prepare your body to deal with things like fear and rage.

This dread can occasionally set off the body's fight-or-flight reaction, resulting in many physiological responses. Get your body ready to either stay and confront the threat or run for safety. Your ability to move fast and make decisions that will increase your chances of success and survival is one way that emotions play an adaptive function.

2. Your Emotions Can Influence Your Decisions

Your emotions significantly impact your decisions, from what you decide to have for breakfast to the candidates you choose to vote for in elections.

Researchers have discovered that persons who suffer from specific kinds of brain injury that impair their capacity for feeling also have lower ability for wise decision-making.

Even when you think logic and reason alone are driving your actions, emotions often play a significant impact. Emotional quotient, or your capacity to understand and manage emotions, has been shown to play an essential role in decision-making.

According to research, fear makes individuals more inclined to perceive risk, disgust makes people more willing to throw away their possessions, and excitement or fury motivates people to take immediate action.

3. Emotions Make You More Comprehensible to Others

Leaving signals while interacting with others is crucial to gauge your emotional state. These signals may include physical manifestations of emotion, such as different facial expressions related to the specific emotions you are feeling.

In other situations, it could entail being honest about your emotions. You are offering others in your life information when you share how you feel, whether it be joy, sadness, excitement, or fear. According to research, happy emotions are felt 2.5 times more frequently than negative ones.

4. Emotions Help You Understand Others

The emotional expressions of individuals around you also provide a plethora of social information, just as your emotions reveal essential information to others.

Being able to recognize and respond to other people's emotions is crucial for effective social communication, which is an essential component of daily living and interpersonal relationships.

It enables you to communicate effectively and create stronger, more meaningful bonds with your friends, family, and other loved ones. Additionally, it allows you to interact with people in various social contexts, such as managing a rowdy employee or a furious client.

Understanding how others express their emotions helps us make sense of them. Understanding how people express their emotions helps us make clear decisions about how to act in a given circumstance.

Controlling your emotions

The next time you are in a circumstance that makes you feel strongly, take a moment to think about the meaning you will give to it. Utilizing one of the following strategies, you can learn to manage your emotions:

1. Breathe deeply

Give yourself some time to think before reacting, whether favorably or adversely.

2. Identify your feelings

"I'm feeling upset because they wounded me," is a simple statement to make. Look farther. Are you upset because you worry they could be correct? Do you feel sad? Emotions are complex and frequently build upon one another.

3. Substitute positive thoughts

Distract yourself if your thoughts immediately turn to how you've been wronged or how awful everything is. Focusing on the good instead of the negative will help you to avoid it. Alter your ideas, and alter your narrative.

4. Manage your energy

Human emotions have enormous strength. Engage in any form of physical activity to release that energy, such as walking, running, or even shooting hoops.

5. Observe your emotions.

Why are you feeling this way? You can learn more about why you're feeling the way you do by keeping a journal or speaking with a trusted friend or family member. It is much simpler to regulate an emotion if you better understand it.

CHAPTER TWO

Managing emotions

Your ideas and feelings can impact your health. Freely experienced and expressed emotions that are unrestricted by attachment or judgment usually flow smoothly without having an adverse effect on our health. Repressed emotions, on the other hand, can drain mental energy, have a detrimental impact on the body, and result in health issues. Being able to experience both pleasant and negative emotions comes naturally to us. Even while we may refer to more challenging emotions as "negative," this does not imply that they are undesirable or that we shouldn't feel them. However, the majority of individuals undoubtedly prefer to experience happy emotions over negative ones. You probably prefer to be joyful than depressed or confident than unsure.

It is crucial to recognize our thoughts and emotions and their impact on our body, conduct, and interpersonal connections.

Negative emotions that are not well-managed are bad for your health.

Chronic stress, which affects the body's hormone balance, depletes the brain chemicals necessary for happiness, and weakens the immune system, can be brought on by negative attitudes and emotions of helplessness and hopelessness. Chronic stress may even lessen our lifespan. The "end caps" of our DNA strands, called telomeres, are shortened by stress, accelerating the aging process (science has recently discovered this).

A wide range of health issues, including hypertension (high blood pressure), cardiovascular illness, digestive problems, and infection, are linked to poorly controlled or suppressed anger (hostility).

Three important ways of managing Emotions

Expressing your feelings

Because they worry about losing control, many people are reluctant to communicate their powerful feelings. This practice can assist you in taking control of your emotions and teaching yourself safe and healthy ways to express them.

- To start, note how you are feeling at this very time.

- Get in the habit of verbally expressing your feelings using "I" language. For instance, I'm feeling terrified, sad, and furious. Respect your feelings.
- Begin by expressing your feelings on your own. Practice with someone you have a secure, trustworthy relationship with once you feel more at ease.
- Finally, start practicing in more difficult circumstances. Do not assign blame to the other person, and be receptive to learning about their experience. You may also get opinions from other people.

Inhale an uplifting thought.

• Breathe in light, love, and healing energy as you inhale into a relaxed abdomen. Think of it as crystal, brilliant, or glittering. As you fill with light and joy, you will notice a brightening inside yourself.

• Completely exhale, letting go of any unfavorable emotions or moods. It may conjure up images of obscurity or a mist. Breathe out any rage, fear, or despair you may be feeling. As you exhale, let any stress, worries, or fears go.

Try the positivity quiz.

We need to be aware of and develop our good traits to counteract our propensity to focus on dangers and other negative feelings. We must be mindful of and nurture our happy feelings. You may live a happier life by learning to recognize positive emotions like joy, amazement, love, appreciation, curiosity, hope, and inspiration.

Five strategies for managing your emotions

1. Self-Care

The pandemic may impede basic functioning due to lack of sleep, increased stress, and loneliness. The secret is to maintain a strong executive function system, which begins with self-care, to have a good connection with your emotions.

Sleep deprivation has been demonstrated to affect self-regulation, which may cause you to have less control over how you react to your emotions. This may explain why you become irritable when you're sleepy. Your bad feelings may keep you awake, creating a vicious cycle that will only make the issue worse.

This can also occur while under stress; thus, a strong stress management strategy can help your executive functions.

So what is the answer? Find things you like to do and include them in your daily routine, such as exercising and keeping a diary.

2. Keep up good relationships.

Having a reliable friend or loved one to confide in also helps us to control our emotions, which is why you normally feel better after venting to a buddy. Making new friends can help you relax your thoughts and even control how your body reacts to emotions. You don't want to shut yourself off from individuals you were close to before, even though we don't get to see each other face to face as frequently as we used to.

3. Stop hiding and start re-evaluating.

The two most researched emotional regulation techniques are called reappraisal and suppression. Suppression is when you try to stop yourself from feeling emotions. When doing this, we frequently discover that unpleasant feelings come back even stronger. Reappraisal is the process of altering the way you see an unpleasant emotion before responding to it.

For instance, if you made a mistake and are dissatisfied, you may remind yourself that it was a teaching moment, increasing the likelihood that your reaction will be positive rather than negative. According to research, this encourages a development attitude, which fosters more positive emotional interactions. The good news is that people may alter their emotional regulation strategies to make them more consistent with reassessment.

4. Practice being aware.

To exercise nonjudgmental awareness, try to meditate. Moreover, it's far more straightforward than you may imagine. You may learn more about your emotional routines by spending only five to ten minutes each day observing how your body and mind feel. This might serve as an exercise for handling emotions in daily life. Pay special attention to any emotions that may occur during your meditation, and follow your gut sense as to how to react.

- What kinds of emotions arise, and how frequently do they occur?
- How do they make you feel physically?
- What happens in your mind?
- When feelings are there, are there any judgments?

Is that answer useful? Is there a more effective way to answer?

5. Avoid emotional explosions.

If you've ever exaggerated a little issue, you undoubtedly felt very horrible afterward. It is thought that routinely practicing prevention is the greatest strategy for handling intense emotional situations.

The issue is that trying to use mindfulness or reappraisal techniques for the first time in a very stressful circumstance is not a good idea.

Avoiding stressful, emotional encounters makes having a good connection with your emotions more likely to make difficult times easier.

Know that it's natural for you not to feel like yourself throughout unexpected moments if you've been having trouble managing your emotions. Don't forget to care for your emotional well-being as we wait for things to return to normal. You may learn to control your emotions by using these tactics to help you unwind, feel good, and stay healthy.

How Bad Emotions Can Be Beneficial

Negative emotions alert us to potential dangers or difficulties that we may have to face. For instance, fear can warn us of potential danger. It serves as a warning that we might need to defend ourselves. Anger alerts us to someone treading on our toes, going over the line, or betraying our trust. Anger may be an indication that we need to defend our own interests.

Our consciousness is focused on negative emotions. They assist us in focusing on an issue so that we may address it. However, experiencing too many unfavorable feelings might leave us overburdened, nervous, worn out, or pressured. Problems may feel insurmountable when negative emotions are out of balance. The more we fixate on unpleasant feelings, the more negative we begin to feel. Focusing on negativity just keeps it going.

How Positive Emotions Can Help Us

Positive emotions counterbalance negative ones, but they also have other potent advantages. Positive emotions alter our brains in ways that broaden our awareness, attention, and memory instead of restricting them, as do negative emotions.

They let us process more information, hold several thoughts simultaneously, and comprehend how various concepts are related to one another.

Positive emotions help us see new possibilities, which makes it easier for us to learn new things and advance our talents. As a result, you perform better on assignments and assessments.

People who experience good emotions are happier, healthier, more intelligent, and socially adept.

The Value of Positive Feelings

Positive feelings are healthy for you and make you feel happy. Pay attention to these practical tools and figure out how to fit them into your daily schedule. Make time in your day for happiness, enjoyment, companionship, rest, thankfulness, and compassion. You'll be happy if you make these things a habit. Here are two facts that can assist us in maximizing the benefits of pleasant emotions:

1. **Allow positive feelings to outweigh negative ones.**

It is simpler to face challenging circumstances when we experience more happy emotions than negative ones.

Our resilience is increased by joyful feelings (the emotional resources needed for coping). They raise our awareness and help us notice additional choices for resolving issues. The negativity bias is a universal human propensity to focus on the bad. The negativity bias predisposes people to focus more on negative than good feelings. When you consider it, it makes sense: Negative emotions draw our attention to issues we may need to address quickly. Negative emotion tuning in may be a survival tactic. However, there is a drawback to the negative bias: It might lead us to believe that a day did not go well, even when we felt both good and terrible feelings. To tip the scales and make a day appear terrific, at least three times as many good feelings are required.

2. Engage in positive behavior daily

We may become happier, perform better, and experience a reduction in our negative emotions by developing behaviors encouraging us to feel better. If we are already coping with a lot of negative emotions like fear, sorrow, anger, irritation, or stress, it is highly crucial to develop good emotions.

Six steps to mastering your emotions

When you first start to feel and experience an emotion entirely is when you should deal with it. In this manner, it won't keep returning repeatedly. These six simple steps will teach you how to regulate your emotions and take charge of your life.

1. **Determine what you actually feel**

Identifying your sentiments is the first step in understanding how to control your emotions. As you go closer to emotional control, consider these questions.

- How do I actually feel right now?
- Do I genuinely feel like...?
- Is there another cause?

2. **Recognize and appreciate your emotions and know that they are there to support you.**

Not suppressing or rejecting your emotions is not the definition of emotional mastery. Instead, learning to control your emotions entails valuing them as an integral part of who you are.

The notion that everything you feel is "wrong" is a fantastic method to sabotage honest communication with yourself and others. You never want to make your emotions incorrect.

3. **Ask yourself what message this emotion is trying to tell you.**

Having emotional control entails engaging your emotions with an inquiry. If you allow them, your feelings will reveal a lot about who you are. Curiosity aids you in:

- Break the emotional cycle you're in.
- Overcome the difficulty;
- Prevent a recurrence of the same issue.

4. **Build confidence**

The easiest and most effective way to gain control of any emotion is to recall a moment when you felt similar emotion and handled it successfully. Since you managed the emotion in the past, surely you can handle it today.

5. **Be confident not only today but also in the future; you can manage this**

Build confidence by practicing addressing circumstances where this feeling could surface in the future if you want to master your emotions. Feel, hear, and perceive how you are managing the circumstance. Doing this, like lifting emotional weights, will develop the "muscle" necessary to manage your emotions properly.

6. Be enthusiastic and act

It's time to celebrate the abilities you now possess since you have learnt to control your emotions.

- Easily manage this feeling;
- Quickly take some action;
- Show that you can manage it.

CHAPTER THREE

What Is The Best Definition Of Ego?

Nowadays, the term "ego" is often used. People readily use it because they think they understand its meaning. However, the phrase is used differently by psychologists and virtual therapists than it is generally.

Depending on how you define ego, it could sound either desirable or something you should want to avoid at all costs. It's both a critical and psychoanalytic phrase. In this piece, we'll examine the word's various interpretations.

Ego is a Latin word that describes one's feeling of self. The ego, often referred to as the self-concept, is a group of ideas that surface when one answers the question, "Who am I?"

These assumptions are characterizations.

In this context, an example of ego would be the remark, "I am an excellent baseball player," which describes one's thoughts about oneself.

Things like sex, nationality, religion, height, weight, skin and eye color, and other distinguishing qualities, might all be viewed as manifestations of the ego.

Since the beliefs are descriptive rather than positive words or feelings—"I feel good about being a terrific baseball player," for instance—it is essential to separate self-concept from self-esteem or self-respect in this context.

Common Definitions of Ego

The term "ego" is sometimes associated with an exaggerated sense of self-importance or self-esteem.

Here are a few instances of how the phrase is typically used:

- We refer to someone as having a huge ego if they think too highly of themselves.
- To describe a group of individuals who may be characterized as conceited or arrogant, we would use the phrase "full of large egos."
- An egomaniac is someone who believes they are superior to and more important than other individuals.

It's important to realize that, despite how it's frequently employed, ego is not inherently negative.

In terms of psychology, ego is more like self-esteem than it is in ordinary speech.

Self-esteem and ego (self-concept) are names for two very separate psychological concepts; however, ego, as used in daily speech, resembles self-esteem more.

Psychological Definition of Ego

The psychological definition of ego differs significantly from the conventional usage of the term. Ego is a term used to define a specific component of oneself in psychology. In essence, it alludes to the conscious mind.

The Self in Relation to Others and the Environment

To distinguish the self from others, psychologists may use the term "ego." Your ego must be intact to differentiate between what you think and what others think. At the core of your ideas, actions, and experiences, your ego communicates with the egos of others you come into contact with outside of yourself.

Perception of Reality

The aspect of you that views reality is known as your ego. You could hear a vehicle honk, taste an apple, or smell a flower. It is your ego that receives and interprets the sensory data. The logical aspect of your intellect is your ego. It makes a note of your surroundings.

Egoism

A philosophical idea is egoism. It's the idea that acting morally always involves looking out for your interests. This may seem absurd to people who believe having a large ego is immoral, yet it's simple to understand why putting yourself first is the wisest course of action. Before attempting to assist another person, airlines advise travelers to put on their own oxygen masks. If you prioritize others too much, you could exhaust yourself, get sick, or experience depression.

Egotism

Having a large ego is the same thing as egotism. You can't quit talking about yourself if you're an egotist. You think you're better and more significant than other people. Since you believe you are the finest, you want everyone to know it.

Egocentrism

The term "egocentrism" was coined by psychologist Jean Piaget to characterize children's incapacity to view the world from a viewpoint other than their own. Later, psychologist David Elkind discussed egocentrism in teens, which he defined as the propensity for adolescents to concentrate on themselves and what other people think of them. "Thinking the world revolves around you" is a frequent expression that accurately describes egocentrism.

What Exactly Does a Healthy Ego Mean?

Both dysfunctional and healthy egos may be distinguished using ego psychology. You have an unrealistic opinion of yourself if you have a weak ego. You can have an inaccurate perception of who you are. You can develop a narcissistic personality or go through a severe depression.

How about a good ego? How does that appear? If your ego is healthy, you typically have positive thoughts about yourself without inflating your accomplishments or skills. You believe your mind is capable of handling the difficulties of life.

You think you are generally decent, respectable, and at least significant to others. Although you can respect other people's viewpoints, your own should always come first.

Ego injury frequently occurs during infancy or in harsh circumstances. Your capacity to regard oneself as valuable might be hampered by what happens to you or what others say about you. You may need to address depression or prior trauma if your ego appears fragile. A therapist can assist you in processing your ideas, emotions, and behaviors to help heal your ego.

What exactly is an ego?

In everyday speech, having a healthy sense of self-respect and self-regard is referred to as having an ego. It's essential to keep in mind that this is not the psychological community's precise definition of ego, which has more to do with how your conscious mind constructs your identity.

An Examination of the Ego

The ego attempts to strike a balance between our moral and idealistic ideals while preventing us from acting on our instinctive cravings (caused by the id) (created by the superego). The ego functions in the preconscious and conscious mind, but because of its close links to the id, it also functions in the unconscious. The reality principle on which the ego is built tries to satiate the impulses d's in a reasonable and acceptable way in society. The ego, for instance, keeps you from chasing after the offending automobile and assaulting the driver if they cut you off in traffic. The ego enables us to see that this reaction would be socially inappropriate while simultaneously allowing us to recognize that there are other, more suitable ways to express our dissatisfaction.

CHAPTER FOUR

How Sleep affects Emotion

Human function and cognition are significantly influenced by sleep, which has an impact on learning, memory, physical recuperation, metabolism, and immunity. It is generally known that sleep serves various purposes in different animals, and more recent studies have shown that sleep also plays a role in controlling emotions. Sleep is essential for both physical and mental health, and managing emotions is key to reducing the negative effects of emotional stress on sleep physiology. Their relationship is mutual.

Our general health and well-being depend on getting enough of the correct sleep. Your body tries to sustain good brain function and preserve physical health while sleeping. Sleep also helps children's and teenagers' bodies and minds grow and develop.

Lack of sleep makes you feel exhausted, makes it difficult to focus and recall things, and may make you cranky.

Additionally, a lack of sleep might affect your judgment and physical coordination. Therefore, having too little sleep impacts how you feel, think, work, learn, and interact with others.

You may need to figure out the cause if you have trouble falling asleep, remaining asleep, or frequently feel exhausted during the day. The good news is that the majority of sleeping issues are easily fixed.

Moods and sleep

Think about how you would feel the following day if you had one restless night or did not get enough sleep. Many of us lack energy, are moody and angry, and have trouble focusing. When things don't go our way, we tend to overreact, and if something positive occurs, we can discover that we don't become as pleased. So it is simple to understand how persistent insomnia might cause concern.

Chronic health issues like diabetes and heart disease are made more likely by a lack of sleep over a long period. Additionally, it has a significant impact on how you feel.

Mood problems and lack of sleep are intimately related. Additionally, it may go both ways: not getting enough sleep can impair your mood and vice versa.

According to studies, persons who lack sleep experience higher levels of negative emotions (such as rage, irritation, impatience, and melancholy) and lower levels of pleasant emotions. Additionally, mood disorders, including despair and anxiety, frequently exhibit sleepiness as a symptom. Additionally, some mental illnesses may be more likely to develop due to it or possibly because of it.

Your emotions can also impact sleep quality. Stress and anxiety cause more agitation and keep your body awake, attentive, and stimulated. You could discover that you cannot shut down your thoughts, that your heart is beating more quickly, and that you are breathing shallowly.

Therefore, receiving the correct kind and amount of sleep is crucial.

How much rest are you requiring?

Your age, degree of physical activity, and overall health influence the amount of sleep you require.

- Teenagers and children should get 9 to 10 hours of sleep per night. Younger kids often go to bed and get up earlier. Teenagers appear to sleep in later and feel weary later than younger kids.
- The average adult needs 8 hours of sleep every night. As we age, we typically require less sleep. These are some broad principles. You could require extra sleep if you (or your children) are exhausted during the day.

Several suggestions for a restful night's sleep

There are several ways you may change your sleeping patterns if you've been experiencing difficulties obtaining enough quality sleep. Try the following advice:

- Establish a regimen and follow it. Attempt to have a consistent bedtime and rise at the same time every day.

- Refrain from consuming alcohol and caffeine too close to bedtime. Additionally, finish eating at least two hours before going to bed.
- Avoid using iPads and TVs in your bedroom.
- Create a refuge in your bedroom. Ensure that your bed is cozy. As you climb into bed, dim the lights. Use the bedroom lamp to read.
- Try basic meditation techniques, such as shutting your eyes for five to ten minutes and concentrating on taking calm, deep breaths.
- Relax in a hot bath.
- Avoid staying up late checking the time. If you are having trouble falling asleep, consider getting up and spending 30 minutes or so reading a book before attempting to do so again.

How does sleep impact the way that positive and negative stimuli are processed?

Sleep is commonly considered significant in how everyday pressures and emotions are processed.

According to scientific research, sleep is crucial for our capacity to manage emotional stress in daily life. It has been discovered that sleep deprivation and insomnia influence social interaction and emotional responsiveness. At several levels of functioning, including the psychomotor, sensory-motor, and cognitive levels, the impact of sleep has been extensively studied; however, the emotional impacts have received less attention.

However, it has been demonstrated that responses to negative emotions are generally greatly amplified, whereas reactions to good events are frequently muted. Research on sleep deprivation discovered that the reaction to positive stimuli was quicker than the reaction brought on by unfavorable and neutral stimuli. Other research has supported this, demonstrating that lack of sleep increases impulsivity toward unpleasant stimuli and subjective ratings of stress, anxiety, and hostility in response to low-stress conditions. Notably, impulsivity is linked to aggressive conduct, a trait related to lack of sleep.

Several mental diseases have sleep disturbances as both a symptom and a risk factor.

Lack of sleep has been linked to higher rates of bewilderment, rage, and sadness, as well as emotions of irritation, aggressiveness, and frustration in research involving children and young people. Subjects saw a rise in psychopathology scores for anxiety, despair, and paranoia even after just one night of sleep deprivation.

Sleep deprivation's long-term impact on mental health

Sleep problems make it difficult to feel happy and can impact the onset and prognosis of affective disorders like depression. The two sleep phases of rapid eye movement (REM) and non-REM (NREM) sleep provide better emotional capacity and adaptability during alertness because both of these sleep phases assist in moderate emotional and motivational impulses. Functional brain activity and adaptive processing are repaired by sound sleep. The integrity of the medial prefrontal cortex-amygdala connections is crucial in regulating emotions. Compared to a typical night of sleep, one night of sleep deprivation causes a 60% increase in the amygdala's response to emotionally disturbing images.

The hormone cortisol's regulatory function, which is involved in regulating stress and responsiveness to emotions, is another important element of regulation. Melatonin is a cause of circadian disruption and explains the change in emotional reactivity and alteration of the circadian cycle as a result of sleep deprivation, which is a source of emotional dysregulation. Melatonin can modulate the response of cortisol.

What does emotional wellness entail?

People with strong emotional health are conscious of their feelings, thoughts, and actions. They now know how to deal with challenges and stress healthily. Stress and troubles are a natural part of life. They have healthy relationships and feel good about themselves.

But a lot of things that occur in your life might disturb your emotional balance and cause uncomfortable emotions like melancholy, tension, or anxiety.

These items consist of:

- Getting fired from your work
- Seeing a child go or come back home
- Coping with a loved one's death
- Divorcing or getting married
- Experiencing a disease or injury
- Securing a promotion at work
- Having financial troubles
- Relocating to a new house
- Having a child

How may my feelings impact my health?

Your thoughts, feelings, and actions affect how your body reacts. It is frequently referred to as the "mind/body link." Your body attempts to alert you to a problem when you are worried, nervous, or unhappy. For instance, a stressful event like losing a loved one may cause high blood pressure or a stomach ulcer. The following physical indicators of unbalanced emotional health include:

- Backache
- Alteration in appetite

- Chest ache
- Diarrhea or constipation
- Mouth dry
- Extreme fatigue
- Aches and pains all over
- Headaches
- Blood pressure problems
- Hypersomnia (trouble sleeping)
- Lightheadedness
- Chest pains (the feeling that your heart is racing)
- Sexual issues
- Breathlessness
- Tense neck
- Sweating
- Stomachache

A weak immune system might make you more susceptible to colds and other diseases when going through emotionally trying periods. Additionally, you might not take care of your health as effectively as you should while feeling pressured, apprehensive, or irritated. It's possible that you don't feel like working out, eating well, or taking the medication your doctor has prescribed. Abuse of other drugs, alcohol, or cigarette products might also point to a problem with one's mental state.

How can I strengthen my emotional well-being?

First, make an effort to identify your feelings and ascertain their causes. Identifying the sources of your life's stress, worry, and unhappiness might help you better manage your emotional well-being. Here are a few other useful hints.

1. **Use the proper language to express your emotions.** Keeping your emotions hidden might make you feel worse if they are tension, unhappiness, or anxiety-related sentiments creating physical issues. Telling your loved ones when something is hurting you is OK. However, bear in mind that your loved ones and friends might not be able to assist you in healthily handling your emotions. Ask someone outside the situation for help during these times, such as your family doctor, a counselor, or a religious leader, for advice and support to help you improve your emotional health.

2. **Keep your life in balance.** Try not to fixate on the issues at work, school, or home that cause unfavorable emotions. This doesn't imply that you should fake happiness when you're pressured, nervous, or sad. While it's vital to deal with these unpleasant emotions, try to keep your attention on the good aspects of your life. You might wish to start a notebook to record the things that bring you joy or tranquility. According to some studies, a cheerful mindset can enhance your quality of life and promote good health. Additionally, you might need to figure out how to let go of certain aspects of your life that are causing you stress and distress. Make time for activities you enjoy.
3. **Become resilient.** Resilient individuals are capable of handling stress in a healthy manner. Various tactics can be used to develop and enhance resilience. Some of these include social support, maintaining a good self-image, embracing change, and maintaining perspective.
4. **Relax your body and mind.** Meditation and other relaxation techniques are effective strategies to regulate your emotions. Guided thinking is a type of meditation.

It can come in a variety of shapes. You can accomplish it, for instance, by working out, stretching, or taking deep breaths. Consult your primary care physician for suggestions on how to unwind.

5. **Ensure your well-being.** It's crucial to take care of your body by following a regular schedule for eating wholesome foods, getting adequate sleep, and exercising to maintain excellent mental health and relieve pent-up tension.
6. **Don't overeat, and don't misuse alcohol or drugs.** Drinking or using drugs just results in further issues, such as family and health issues.

Being conscious of your thoughts, feelings, and actions is the first step toward having good emotional health. It's natural to develop coping mechanisms for stress and issues as you go through life. It's crucial to feel good about yourself and have positive connections.

Your emotional well-being can be affected by a variety of life events. Strong emotions of melancholy, worry, or anxiety may result from them. Unwanted changes may be just as stressful as positive or desired changes.

Your thoughts, feelings, and actions affect how your body reacts. One example of a "mind/body link" is this. Your body responds physiologically when you're worried, nervous, or disturbed. After a traumatic incident, such as losing a loved one, you can experience high blood pressure or a stomach ulcer.

CHAPTER FIVE

Ways to Getting Better Health

There are methods for enhancing emotional well-being. Recognize your feelings and the reasons behind them first. Identifying the sources of your life's stress, worry, and unhappiness might help you better manage your emotional well-being. Here are a few other useful hints.

Use the proper language to express your emotions.

Keeping your emotions hidden might make you feel worse if they are tension, unhappiness, or anxiety-related sentiments that are creating physical issues. Telling your loved ones when something is hurting you is OK. But remember that your loved ones might not always be able to support you in handling your emotions correctly. Ask someone outside the situation for assistance at these moments. To assist you in enhancing your mental health, consider consulting a family physician, a psychotherapist, or a religious leader.

Keep your life in balance.

Pay attention to the aspects of your life for which you are thankful. Try not to fixate on the issues at work, school, or home that lead to negative feelings. This does not imply that you should fake happiness when you're pressured, nervous, or sad. While dealing with bad emotions is necessary, try to keep your attention on the good aspects of your life as well. You might wish to start a notebook to record the things that bring you joy or tranquility. A cheerful mindset can enhance your quality of life and promote good health. Additionally, you might need to figure out how to let go of certain aspects of your life that are causing you stress and distress. Make time to do the activities you like.

Become resilient.

Resilient individuals are better at constructively managing stress. You may learn to be resilient and reinforced through various tactics. These include having a strong social network, maintaining a good self-image, embracing change, and maintaining perspective. With cognitive behavioral therapy, a therapist or counselor can assist you in achieving this objective (CBT). If this is a good idea for you, ask your doctor.

Relax your body and mind.

Your emotions can be balanced by using relaxation techniques like yoga, Tai Chi, guided visualization, guided meditation, and listening to music. YouTube also offers free guided imagery films. Guided thinking is a type of meditation. It can come in a variety of shapes. For instance, you may accomplish it by moving about, stretching, or taking deep breaths. Consult your primary care physician for suggestions on how to unwind.

Ensure your own well-being.

It's essential to take good care of your body by following a regular schedule if you want to maintain good mental health. Establish a schedule of good food, rest, and exercise to release tension. Don't overeat, and don't misuse alcohol or drugs. Drinking or using drugs leads to further difficulties, such as family and health troubles.

Things to Think About

Your body's immune system might be compromised by poor mental wellness. You are more susceptible to getting colds and other diseases when going through emotionally trying times.

Additionally, you might not take care of your health as effectively as you should while you're feeling pressured, apprehensive, or irritated. It's possible that you don't feel like working out, eating well, or taking the medication your doctor has prescribed. You could misuse other medicines, alcohol, or cigarettes.

How emotions affects health

Living under chronic danger has detrimental effects on one's health.

1. **Physical well-being.** Fear impairs our immune system, weakens the heart, and increases the risk of ulcers, irritable bowel syndrome, and diminished fertility. It may cause early mortality or even hastened aging.
2. **Memory.** Long-term memory development can be hindered by fear and harm some brain regions, including the hippocampus. Due to this, managing fear may become even more challenging, and a person may become nervous most of the time. Someone who experiences chronic anxiety perceives the world as dangerous, and their memories support this.

3. **Reactivity and processing in the brain.** Fear can all interfere with our ability to control our emotions, understand nonverbal signs and other indications, contemplate before acting, and behave morally. This has a detrimental effect on our thinking and decision-making, making us more prone to intense emotions and impulsive behaviors. All of these impacts may prevent us from acting as we should.

Mental wellness Fatigue, severe depression, and PSTD are other effects of long-term dread. Threats to our security, therefore, affect our emotional and physical welfare, whether they are genuine or perceived.

The Best Way to Take Control of Your Emotions

You might be surprised to learn how vital it is to have the capacity to feel and express emotions.

Emotions are a significant factor in your reactions since they represent your emotional response to a circumstance. When you're in tune with them, you have access to crucial information that supports: decision-making, successful relationships; daily interactions; and self-care.

While emotions can be beneficial in daily life, when they feel out of control, they can have a negative impact on your emotional well-being and interpersonal connections.

To get you started, consider the following advice.

1. **Consider the effect of your emotions.**

Not all strong emotions are negative. Emotions give our life excitement, individuality, and vibrancy. Strong emotions may indicate that we completely embrace life and aren't suppressing our innate responses.

Therefore, take some time to evaluate how your irrational emotions impact your daily life. Problem regions will be simpler to spot as a result (and track your success).

2. **Opt for regulation rather than suppression**

If it were that simple to regulate your emotions, you could do it with a dial. But consider for a second that you could control your emotions in this manner.

You wouldn't want to leave them operating at full capacity constantly. You wouldn't want to turn them off either completely.

You restrict yourself from feeling and expressing emotions when you suppress or repress them. This may occur intentionally (suppression) or unintentionally (repression).

Both mental and physical health symptoms, such as anxiety, sadness, problems sleeping, discomfort in the muscles, and difficulties concentrating, can be influenced by either.

Make sure you aren't just brushing your emotions under the rug while you are trying to regulate them. It's important to strike a balance between having too many feelings and having none at all for healthy emotional expression.

3. Recognize your emotions.

You may start taking back control by taking a moment to check in with your emotions.

Let's say you've been dating someone for a while. You attempted to set up a date with them last week, but they declined. You contacted me again yesterday with the message, "I'd want to meet you soon. Are you available this week?

After more than a day, they finally respond: "Can't. Busy."

All of a sudden, you're pretty upset. You kick your wastebasket, throw your phone across the room, and kick your desk, stubbing your toe.

Asking yourself, "What am I feeling right now?" will interrupt you. (displeased, perplexed, and enraged) • What has happened to cause me to feel this way? (They ignored me without explaining.)

- Is there any explanation for the circumstance that would make sense? (Perhaps they're under stress, ill, or coping with another issue that they don't feel comfortable disclosing. They could want to provide further details when they can.)
- What do I want to do in response to these emotions? (Scream, toss things in anger, and send an offensive text back.)
- Is there a more effective method to handle them? (Ask whether all is well. Question their upcoming availability. Take a stroll or a run.)

You can change your first extreme response by reframing your thinking to consider potential alternatives.

It could take some time before this reaction gets ingrained in you. Practice will make it simpler to do these actions (and more effective) mentally.

4. Accept all of your feelings.

Try downplaying your feelings to yourself if you want to improve your ability to control your emotions.

It may seem beneficial to tell yourself, "Just calm down," or "It's not that big of an issue, so don't stress out," when you start to hyperventilate after hearing wonderful news or collapse on the floor weeping and shouting when you can't locate your keys.

However, this discredits your experience. To you, it is really important. You can become more at ease with your emotions if you accept them as they are. Getting more at ease with solid feelings enables you to fully feel them without reacting in extreme, unhelpful ways.

Try viewing emotions as messengers to learn to accept them. They are neither nice nor bad. They are impartial. Even though they occasionally trigger negative emotions, they still provide helpful information.

5. Maintain a mood diary

Putting your emotions and the reactions they elicit into writing (or typing) might help you identify any disruptive patterns.

Sometimes it's sufficient to follow your thoughts back via your emotions mentally. Writing down emotions might help you think about them more thoroughly.

It also aids in identifying the situations that lead to emotions that are more difficult to manage, such as difficulties at work or family conflicts. Finding precise triggers enables the development of more effective management techniques.

When you journal every day, it is extremely beneficial. Keep a diary close by and record strong feelings or emotions as they arise. Try to keep track of your reaction and the triggers. If your response wasn't helpful, utilize your diary to research further potential solutions that could.

6. Inhale deeply.

The strength of a deep breath has a lot to offer, whether you're exuberantly joyful or utterly furious.

Even if that's not the intention, slowing down and focusing on your breathing won't make the feelings disappear.

However, practicing deep breathing can help you center yourself and take a step back from the initial, overwhelming emotion and any excessive reaction you'd want to avoid.

When your emotions start to overtake you in the future:

- Inhale gradually. The diaphragm, not the chest, is where deep breaths originate. Visualizing your breath rising from your abdomen may be of assistance.
- Retain it. Breathe in for three counts, then gently let it out.
- Think about a mantra. Some people believe that repeating a mantra, such as "I am tranquil," I am calm," or "I am relaxed."

7. Recognize when to use your voice

Everything has its own time and place, including strong emotions. For instance, crying uncontrollably after losing a loved one is a typical reaction. After getting dumped, screaming or even beating your pillow may help you release some tension and fury.

However, in other circumstances, some restraint is required. No matter how angry you are about an unfair disciplinary action, yelling at your supervisor won't solve the problem.

You may learn when it's OK to express your sentiments and when you might want to sit with them for the time being by being aware of your surroundings and the scenario.

8. Make room for yourself

Keeping your emotions at bay might help you ensure that you're rationally responding to them. Physical separation, such as leaving a distressing circumstance, might constitute this distance. But by diverting your attention, you may also establish some mental space.

It's not healthy to completely ignore or avoid feelings, but it's also OK to divert your attention from them until you're in a better position to deal with them. Just be sure to revisit them. Healthy diversion only lasts for a short time. Take a stroll, watch a hilarious video, have a conversation with a loved one, or spend some time with your pet.

9. Attempt meditation

It could be one of your go-to strategies for handling intense emotions if you already meditate. You may become more conscious of all emotions and sensations by practicing meditation.

When you practice meditation, you're training yourself to be aware of such emotions, to acknowledge them without condemning or trying to modify or suppress them.

Emotional control may be made simpler by learning to accept all of your feelings, as was already indicated. You may improve these accepting abilities by meditating. Other advantages include improving your ability to unwind and sleep better.

You may get started by reading our guide on the many types of meditation.

10. Manage your stress well

It might be challenging to control your emotions when you're under a lot of stress. Even those who typically have good emotional self-control may find it more difficult to do so in extreme stress and anxiety conditions.

Your emotions can become more controllable by reducing stress or learning more effective stress management techniques.

Mindfulness techniques, such as meditation, can help with stress, too. They won't eliminate it, but they can make it more bearable.

Making time for leisure and hobbies, getting adequate sleep, talking and laughing with friends, exercising, and spending time in nature are all good methods to manage stress.

11. Consult a counselor

If your feelings are still too much for you to handle, it might be time to get professional help.

Several mental health illnesses, including bipolar disorder and borderline personality disorder, are associated with long-term or persistent emotional dysregulation and mood swings. Having trouble managing your emotions might also be related to trauma, familial problems, or other underlying difficulties.

A therapist can provide understanding, judgment-free assistance while you:

- Investigate the causes of dysregulated emotions.
- Manage extreme mood swings.
- Learn how to down-regulate intense feelings or up-regulate limited emotional expression.

Swings in mood and strong emotions might bring undesirable or negative ideas, which can eventually bring on feelings of helplessness or despair.

This loop may eventually result in unproductive coping mechanisms like self-harm or suicidal thoughts. Speak to a loved one you can trust if you start to experience suicidal thoughts or desire to hurt yourself so they can assist you and receive support immediately away.

CONCLUSION

Emotional mastery is one of the most effective abilities you can develop to have an authentic and satisfying life.

In suggestions regarding emotion, the concepts of arousal, motivation, reinforcement, and emotion frequently coexist. The ability to approach phenomena connected to emotion, motivation, reinforcement and arousal as parts of a cohesive process occurs when an organism encounters a problem or an opportunity that comes from a focus on survival functions and circuits.

Positive thinking has both physiological and psychological advantages, such as quicker recovery from cardiovascular stress, better sleep, fewer colds, and an increased sense of general satisfaction. The good news is that positive attitudes, such as playfulness, appreciation, amazement, love, curiosity, calm, and a sense of connection to others, not only have an immediate influence.

www.ingramcontent.com/pod-product-compliance
Lightning Source LLC
LaVergne TN
LVHW052100160826
845678LV00015B/3301

* 9 7 9 8 3 5 1 7 6 2 2 5 8 *